HERBAL REMEDIES FOR SKIN CANCER PREVENTION

A Beginner's Guide to Learn Simple Herbal Practices to Safeguard Your Skin from the Risks of Skin Cancer

DR. CHRIS FRIEDRICH

Skin cancer prevention is a major global health concern, and increasing incidence rates call for a thorough understanding and preventative measures. Herbal Remedies for Skin Cancer Prevention" is an invaluable guide that addresses a critical gap in health literature by emphasizing the holistic approach to protecting against skin cancer. The book's goal is multifaceted, encompassing education, empowerment, and practical application of herbal remedies in the context of skin cancer prevention.

Given the potentially fatal effects of unchecked progression, the importance of preventing skin cancer cannot be overstated. This book provides a thorough overview of the types, causes, and risk factors of skin cancer, highlighting the critical role of prevention and the significance of incorporating herbal remedies into daily life to strengthen the body's natural defenses.

An important part of the book explores the history of herbal remedies and their benefits for preventing skin cancer.

Readers learn about the variety of herbal allies that are available, such as immune-stimulating herbs like garlic and echinacea, skin-healing herbs like aloe vera and calendula, and antioxidant-rich herbs like green tea and turmeric.

Beyond herbal remedies, the book advocates for lifestyle changes critical to skin health, stress management, sun protection, a nourishing diet, and regular exercise. It also provides helpful advice on herbal preparations, from infusions and teas to tinctures, salves, and balms.

Through case studies and success stories, practical application is brought to life, offering concrete proof of the effectiveness of herbal remedies; additionally, the book delves into the integration of herbal remedies with conventional approaches, promoting cooperation with medical professionals and providing insights into complementary therapies.

Common questions about herbal remedies for skin cancer prevention are answered with evidence-based answers, and readers are guided through the process of creating personalized herbal skincare routines with an emphasis on monitoring and adjusting for optimal results.

"Herbal Remedies for Skin Cancer Prevention" is a beacon of knowledge, empowering readers to take proactive steps towards skin health through informed choices and the incorporation of herbal wisdom into their daily lives. The book culminates in a valuable repository of resources and references, including websites, organizations, books, and scientific studies that are recommended.

Introduction

Herbal remedies, with their roots in traditional knowledge and the abundance of nature, offer a promising avenue for preventing skin cancer and maintaining skin health. The investigation of herbal remedies for skin cancer prevention is an important undertaking in the field of holistic health and well-being. Given the increasing global incidence of skin cancer, it is imperative to explore alternative approaches that can supplement conventional methods. The search for effective preventive measures is motivated by the same desire to support natural and sustainable healthcare practices.

The objective of the Book:

This book aims to provide a valuable resource for people looking for natural ways to protect their skin from the risk of cancer.

It unravels the potential of herbal remedies in the prevention of skin cancer through a thorough examination of various herbs, their active compounds, and their historical use in traditional medicine.

It also serves as a guide for those interested in incorporating herbal solutions into their skincare routine, emphasizing preventive strategies that harness the power of nature to support overall skin health.

The significance of preventing skin cancer

In the context of public health and individual well-being, it is critical to recognize the significance of skin cancer prevention. Skin cancer, which includes melanoma, basal cell carcinoma, and squamous cell carcinoma, poses serious health risks and can have severe consequences if left untreated. Prevention becomes essential not only to avoid the psychological and physical toll that cancer takes but also to lessen the strain on healthcare systems. Herbal remedies, with their potential protective properties, provide a means of empowering individuals to take proactive measures toward skin cancer prevention, thereby contributing to overall health outcomes.

Synopsis of Herbal Treatments

This section of the book explores the variety of herbs, their extracts, and formulations that have shown promise in scientific studies or have been traditionally used for skin care. From aloe vera and calendula to green tea and turmeric, the reader will gain insights into the multifaceted benefits of these herbal remedies.

The overview also emphasizes the importance of considering these remedies as complementary to established preventive measures, fostering a holistic approach to skin cancer prevention that integrates conventional and alternative practices. Overall, a broad range of plant-based interventions that have historically been recognized for their skin-nourishing and protective properties are covered by the overview of herbal remedies.

CHAPTER 1
UNDERSTANDING SKIN CANCER

Melanoma, squamous cell carcinoma, and basal cell carcinoma are the three primary forms of skin cancer. Each type has different characteristics and severity; basal cell carcinoma is the most common and least aggressive form, while squamous cell carcinoma is more aggressive and may spread to other areas of the body. Melanoma, though less common, is the most deadly form, often spreading rapidly if not detected early. Skin cancer is a common and potentially life-threatening condition that arises from the abnormal growth of skin cells. Understanding the various types of skin cancer is essential to effectively address prevention strategies.

Reasons and Danger Factors

To develop preventive measures, it is necessary to understand the causes of skin cancer as well as the risk factors that contribute to the disease's development. Long-term exposure to UV radiation from the sun or tanning beds is one of the main risk factors, along with a history of sunburns, fair skin, weakened immune systems, and a family history of the disease. Additionally, exposure to certain chemicals and substances, like arsenic and certain industrial compounds, may increase the risk of developing skin cancer. By identifying these factors, individuals can make educated lifestyle choices to lower their risk of developing skin cancer.

The Value of Prevention

In addition to regular skin examinations, the use of herbal remedies has garnered attention for its potential role in preventing skin cancer.

These natural alternatives often contain compounds with antioxidant and anti-inflammatory properties, which may help protect the skin from damage and reduce the risk of cancer development.

However, it is important to approach herbal remedies cautiously and consult with healthcare professionals. Prevention is key to lowering the incidence of skin cancer and promoting overall skin health. Given the known risk factors, adopting sun protection measures is paramount.

This includes using sunscreen with a high SPF, wearing protective clothing, and seeking shade during peak sunlight hours.

Ultimately, a thorough comprehension of skin cancer, including its types, causes, and risk factors, emphasizes the importance of prevention. Including herbal remedies and protective measures in a holistic approach to skin health may help lower the incidence of skin cancer. By raising awareness and implementing preventive measures, people can take control of their skin health and reduce the risks that may arise from this common condition.

CHAPTER 2

HERBAL APPROACHES TO THE PREVENTION OF SKIN CANCER

In contrast to conventional medical interventions that frequently involve surgery, radiation, and chemotherapy, the herbal approach to skin cancer prevention is a holistic and alternative perspective that tackles the increasing global incidence of skin cancers.

It is based on the idea that nature has a multitude of compounds that can work in concert to prevent the initiation and progression of skin cancers; the emphasis is not only on treating symptoms but also on addressing the underlying causes and promoting overall skin health.

This shift in thinking towards herbal remedies is in line with the growing interest in natural and sustainable healthcare practices.

An Historical View on Herbal Medicines

The historical perspective on herbal remedies for preventing skin cancer reveals a rich tapestry of traditional knowledge and practices that have been passed down through the generations.

Herbs have been revered for their medicinal properties across cultures and civilizations, and one of their potential uses is preventing skin cancer.

Certain herbs have been used for promoting skin health and preventing malignancies, according to ancient healing systems like Ayurveda, Traditional Chinese Medicine, and indigenous practices. Historical texts and ethnobotanical records offer insights into the complex relationship between nature and healthcare in various societies.

The benefits of using herbal remedies

Beyond their historical origins, herbal remedies offer several benefits that set them apart from conventional approaches to skin cancer prevention. Most notably, herbal remedies have the potential to have fewer side effects than synthetic drugs; many have a gentler profile, which minimizes adverse reactions that are typically associated with chemotherapy and other aggressive treatments; herbs also often contain a complex mixture of bioactive compounds, which allows for a multitargeted approach that addresses various pathways involved in cancer development; this inherent complexity offers a robust defense against cancer cells and supports the body's natural ability to maintain balance, providing a more complex and all-encompassing approach to skin cancer prevention.

Using Herbs in Everyday Life

Herbs can be incorporated into daily routines through a variety of means, such as culinary use, herbal teas, topical applications, and supplements. Understanding the optimal dosage, preparation methods, and potential interactions is crucial for effective integration.

Additionally, fostering awareness about the benefits of specific herbs for skin health can empower individuals to make informed decisions in their daily lives. This shift towards preventive herbal practices not only contributes to skin cancer prevention but also promotes overall well-being and a harmonious relationship among people.

As a whole, the herbal approach to skin cancer prevention is a complex strategy that combines traditional knowledge with contemporary understanding. Researching the historical origins of herbal remedies reveals a wealth of information that cuts across cultural divides.

The benefits of herbal remedies, such as their potential for fewer side effects and multitargeted action, make them promising allies in the fight against skin cancer. Including herbs in daily life necessitates a holistic approach that emphasizes the value of proactive decisions and a symbiotic relationship with nature. As this field of study advances, the herbal approach is poised to make a substantial contribution to the changing landscape of cancer prevention by providing a natural and sustainable option.

CHAPTER 3
IDENTIFYING HERBAL ALLIES

The potential role of herbal remedies in preventing skin cancer has garnered attention in recent years. Developing effective preventive strategies requires understanding the properties of various herbs and how they affect skin health. Three categories of herbs have shown promise through extensive research: antioxidant-rich herbs, immune-boosting herbs, and skin-healing herbs.

Rich in antioxidant herbs

Free radicals are extremely reactive molecules that can damage DNA and other cellular structures. Green tea is one powerful antioxidant-rich herb that has received a lot of attention. Green tea contains polyphenols, especially epigallocatechin gallate (EGCG), which have strong antioxidant properties.

Studies have shown that drinking green tea regularly can protect the skin from UV radiation damage and lower the risk of developing skin cancer.

Another noteworthy antioxidant-rich herb is turmeric, which also contains curcumin, a compound known for its anti-inflammatory and antioxidant effects. Studies have looked into the potential of curcumin in treating and preventing cancer, including skin cancer.

 Curcumin is a valuable herbal ally in the prevention of skin cancer because it can modulate molecular pathways involved in the development of cancer.

The anti-inflammatory and antimicrobial qualities of rosemary contribute to its protective effects on the skin. Adding rosemary to skincare routines or eating it as part of a balanced diet may offer additional defense against skin cancer.

Rosemary is known for its high content of Rosmarinus acid and other antioxidants, which may help prevent skin cancer.

Anti-Immune Herbs

Echinacea, a well-known immune-boosting herb, has been traditionally used to support the immune system. Its immunomodulatory effects involve enhancing the activity of various immune cells. While further research is necessary to establish a direct link between echinacea and skin cancer prevention, the herb's potential to bolster overall immune function is a promising avenue for exploration. A robust immune system is integral to the body's ability to detect and eliminate abnormal cells, including those that may lead to skin cancer.

Another immune-stimulating herb with deep roots in traditional Chinese medicine, astragalus, has drawn interest for its possible cancer-preventive qualities. Research indicates that astragalus may strengthen the body's defense mechanisms, increasing its capacity to identify and eradicate potentially cancerous cells. Adding astragalus to dietary or supplement regimens could strengthen the immune system as part of a comprehensive strategy to prevent skin cancer.

Though more research specifically addressing skin cancer prevention is necessary, garlic's general impact on immune function positions it as a valuable ally in the pursuit of holistic skin health. Garlic is widely known for its antimicrobial and immune-modulating properties, but it also stands out as an immune-boosting herb with potential implications for skin cancer prevention. Allicin, a compound found in garlic, has been studied for its anti-cancer effects.

Herbs that Heal Skin

Supporting the skin's natural healing processes is just as important as preventing skin cancer. Aloe vera, a well-known herb that heals skin, has been used for centuries to soothe and aid in the healing of a variety of skin conditions. Packed with vitamins, minerals, and polysaccharides, aloe vera helps to reduce inflammation and helps damaged skin cells regenerate. When applied topically, aloe vera may provide a protective barrier against harmful environmental factors, which may lower the risk of skin cancer.

Calendula has been studied for its potential in wound healing and skin regeneration. Its anti-inflammatory and antimicrobial qualities are well-known. Flavonoids, which are present in calendula, contribute to its antioxidant effects and support its role in preventing skin cancer. Adding calendula to skincare routines or using it in topical formulations may provide extra layers of protection for the skin.

Allantoin, a compound found in comfrey, promotes cell proliferation and tissue repair. While research on comfrey's specific role in skin cancer prevention is limited, its traditional use in promoting skin health suggests potential benefits when used judiciously. Comfrey has been used historically for its skin-healing properties, although it should be used cautiously due to potential liver toxicity concerns.

finding herbal allies to help prevent skin cancer requires a sophisticated understanding of the properties of different herbs and how they work. For example, antioxidant-rich herbs like green tea, turmeric, and rosemary help protect the skin from oxidative stress by neutralizing free radicals; immune-boosting herbs like echinacea, astragalus, and garlic support the body's defense mechanisms and may help identify and eliminate abnormal cells; and skin-healing herbs like aloe vera, calendula, and comfrey are vital for promoting the skin's natural healing processes. Although these herbal remedies show promise, it is important to use them in conjunction with other preventative measures like sun protection, a healthy lifestyle, and routine medical care.

CHAPTER 4
HERBAL READYMADE

Herbal preparations are a mainstay of traditional medicine and have been used for centuries due to their therapeutic properties in many cultures. When it comes to preventing skin cancer, using herbal preparations is a natural and holistic approach. Many different types of herbal preparations are used, and each one has a specific purpose in promoting skin health and possibly lowering the risk of skin cancer.

Teas and Infusions

One of the most popular and easily obtained herbal preparations is infusions and teas. Infusions are made by steeping medicinal herbs in hot water to release their beneficial compounds. This process aids in the absorption of bioactive components, such as antioxidants and polyphenols, which support skin health.

Several herbs that are known to have anti-cancer properties, like turmeric (Curcuma longa), green tea (Camellia sinensis), and calendula (Calendula officinalis), can be used in infusions. These herbal teas are a delightful way to include medicinal plants in one's routine, and they may also offer a potential means of preventing skin cancer through regular consumption.

Tinctures

In the context of skin cancer prevention, tinctures can be made from herbs with anti-inflammatory and antioxidant properties, such as echinacea (Echinacea purpureal), aloe vera (Aloe barbadensis), and chamomile (Matric aria chamomilla). Regular application of herbal tinctures to the skin may provide a protective barrier and promote overall skin health, potentially lowering the risk of skin cancer development. Tinctures are made from dried herbs using alcohol or other solvents, yielding a concentrated liquid form of the medicinal constituents that is easy to administer and absorb.

Balms and Salves

A topical approach to herbal skin care, salves, and balms combine the benefits of medicinal herbs with skin-nourishing oils and waxes to create a protective layer on the skin that helps retain moisture and delivers herbal compounds. Commonly included herbs in salves and balms are calendula, comfrey (Symphytum officinal), and lavender (Lavandula angustifolia) for their regenerative and soothing qualities; regular application of such herbal formulations may prevent skin cancer by enhancing skin integrity and resilience.

Apply Poultices

Herbs with anti-inflammatory and wound-healing properties, like aloe vera, plantain (Plantago major), and turmeric, can be used in poultices for potential skin cancer prevention.

The localized application of herbal poultices may aid in reducing inflammation, supporting tissue repair, and enhancing the overall health of the skin in specific areas of concern. Poultices are a way to apply ground or mashed herbs directly onto the skin, creating a localized herbal compress that is applied directly onto the skin.

Herbal Soaps

Herbal baths are a unique and soothing way to incorporate medicinal herbs into a skincare routine. By adding herbs that are known for their skin-nourishing and therapeutic properties to bathwater, people can benefit from a holistic approach to skin cancer prevention. Popular choices for herbal baths include rosemary (Rosmarinus officinalis), chamomile, and calendula. Regular herbal baths may improve overall skin health by reducing the risk of developing skin cancer through the combination of relaxation, hydration, and absorption of herbal extracts.

The use of herbal preparations to prevent skin cancer involves a variety of formulations, each with its benefits. From the easily accessed and enjoyable herbal teas to the focused and external application of salves and poultices, these preparations provide a comprehensive strategy for enhancing skin health. The addition of medicinal herbs with established anti-inflammatory, antioxidant, and wound-healing qualities offers a natural way for people to actively participate in their skin cancer prevention plans.

As with any health approach, seeking the advice of a healthcare provider is necessary to make sure that herbal preparations are in line with one's specific health needs and work in conjunction with current medical interventions.

CHAPTER 5

MODIFYING LIFESTYLE TO PROMOTE SKIN HEALTH

One of the most important ways to prevent skin cancer is to maintain healthy skin through lifestyle modifications. These changes should be comprehensive and include sun protection, a healthy diet, stress management, and regular exercise. Since the skin is the largest organ in the body and is responsible for protecting it from outside threats, it is important to adopt practices that improve its general health. Lifestyle modifications can lower the risk of skin cancer and improve skin health in general.

The Value of Sun Protection

To prevent skin cancer, sun protection is crucial because prolonged exposure to ultraviolet (UV) radiation is a major risk factor. UV rays from the sun can damage skin cells' DNA, causing mutations that may contribute to the development of cancer. Regular use of sunscreen with a high SPF, along with wearing protective clothing and finding shade during the hours of maximum sunlight, are important ways to reduce the risks associated with UV radiation exposure. Awareness of the benefits of sun protection and adoption of these practices can help.

A Good Diet to Prevent Skin Cancer

A balanced and nutrient-dense diet is important for overall health and plays a major role in preventing skin cancer. Some nutrients and antioxidants found in fruits, vegetables, and other wholesome foods have been linked to skin health and protection. Including a diet high in vitamins, minerals, and antioxidants may also help strengthen the skin's defense mechanisms against environmental factors, such as UV radiation.

Foods with anti-inflammatory properties may also help reduce inflammation, which is one of the factors that contribute to the development of skin cancer.

Stress Reduction

Stress can worsen inflammation and impair the body's ability to repair damaged DNA, which may increase the risk of developing cancer. Adopting stress-reducing practices like mindfulness, meditation, and relaxation techniques can positively impact overall health and contribute to the prevention of skin cancer. The complex relationship between stress and skin health highlights the importance of stress management in skin cancer prevention. Chronic stress can negatively affect the immune system, making the body more susceptible to various health issues, including skin cancer.

Frequent Workout

Regular physical activity is linked to improved circulation, which can enhance the delivery of nutrients and oxygen to the skin, aiding in its maintenance and repair. It is also associated with the regulation of various hormones and growth factors that influence skin health. Keeping up a regular exercise routine is a proactive measure that complements other lifestyle changes in preventing skin cancer and promoting overall skin vitality. Physical activity is an essential part of a healthy lifestyle and plays a significant role in protecting against skin cancer.

In conclusion, modifying one's lifestyle is essential to preventing skin cancer. A comprehensive strategy includes sun protection, a balanced diet, stress reduction, and regular exercise. Knowing the importance of each of these factors and implementing them into one's daily routine can improve skin health overall and lower the risk of developing skin cancer. Adopting these practices necessitates dedication to long-term routines that put skin health first, reflecting a holistic approach to cancer prevention that takes into account both physical and mental well-being.

CHAPTER 6
CASE STUDIES AND SUCCESS STORIES

In the field of herbal remedies for the prevention of skin cancer, case studies and success stories are invaluable tools for comprehending the potential effectiveness of alternative treatments.

These accounts offer a thorough analysis of people who have included herbal remedies in their preventive strategies, illuminating the results and experiences they encountered. By examining these cases, researchers and practitioners gain insight into the various approaches people have taken, enabling a thorough analysis of the practical applications of herbal remedies.

Case studies not only highlight successful outcomes but also any difficulties or constraints encountered, adding to a nuanced understanding of the complexities surrounding herbal interventions.

Actual Herbal Medicine Experiences

Examining real-life accounts of people who have chosen herbal remedies as part of their preventive measures reveals a rich tapestry of individual journeys in skin cancer prevention. These narratives delve into the personal accounts of people who have made this decision and analyze these experiences by looking at the particular herbs used, the length of the regimen, lifestyle changes, and any concurrent conventional treatments. Understanding why people choose herbal remedies also offers important insights into the factors that influence decision-making in skin cancer prevention. Finally, a nuanced examination of these real-life experiences leads to a comprehensive understanding of the complex nature of herbal interventions and their effects on individuals.

Before and Following

Examining before-and-after stories can help establish correlations between particular herbal formulations and observable outcomes, which is valuable information for evidence-based decision-making in skin cancer prevention.

Before-and-after stories typically include thorough documentation of the condition before the initiation of herbal interventions and subsequent improvements observed over time.

The stories enable practitioners and researchers to visually assess changes in skin health, lesion size, and overall well-being. Additionally, photographs are frequently included in these accounts, adding a tangible dimension to the evaluation of herbal remedies.

A lesson discovered

To improve future methods and interventions, the lessons learned from the application of herbal remedies in the prevention of skin cancer must be explored. This entails a thoughtful examination of both successful and unsuccessful cases to spot trends, similarities, and variables that influence the results. The lessons learned cover a wide range of topics, such as the choice of herbs, dosage, length of treatment, individual differences, and potential interactions with conventional medicine. By combining these insights, practitioners can improve their comprehension of the subtleties surrounding herbal interventions, allowing for more customized and informed recommendations. Furthermore, by identifying potential pitfalls and challenges, they help to build a growing body of knowledge.

Lessons learned from these experiences form the foundation for refining future approaches, ensuring a more informed and evidence-based approach to herbal interventions for skin cancer prevention. In summary, case studies and success stories provide a detailed exploration of the real-world applications of herbal remedies, offering valuable insights into their efficacy and challenges. Real-life experiences highlight the diverse approaches individuals take in incorporating herbal remedies into their preventive strategies, contributing to a nuanced understanding of the complexities involved. Before-and-after stories provide visual and anecdotal evidence of the impact of herbal remedies on skin health, aiding in the assessment of their effectiveness.

CHAPTER 7
INTEGRATING HERBAL REMEDIES WITH CONVENTIONAL APPROACHES

Combining the benefits of herbal remedies—which are often derived from plants and other natural sources—with conventional approaches in the prevention of skin cancer is a complex and multifaceted approach to holistic healthcare. Conventional approaches, on the other hand, include medical interventions like radiation therapy, chemotherapy, and surgery.

The combination of these two paradigms can provide a comprehensive strategy that tackles the complexities of skin cancer prevention.

By combining the strengths of herbal remedies—which have inherent bioactive compounds—and the rigor of conventional medical practices, a more robust and effective preventive approach can be achieved.

Working together with medical professionals

The collaboration between individuals seeking herbal remedies for skin cancer prevention and healthcare professionals is paramount in ensuring a balanced and evidence-based approach. Healthcare professionals, including dermatologists and oncologists, play a crucial role in guiding patients through preventive measures. The integration of herbal remedies into the dialogue between patients and healthcare providers requires open communication, mutual understanding, and a shared commitment to patient well-being. Professionals can provide valuable insights into the potential benefits and risks associated with specific herbal remedies, taking into account individual patient profiles, existing health conditions, and potential interactions with conventional treatments.

This collaborative approach fosters an environment where patients are empowered to make informed decisions about incorporating herbal remedies into their skin cancer prevention strategies while benefiting from the expertise of medical professionals.

Alternative Medicines

Complementary therapies recognize the interconnectedness of various approaches, acknowledging that a holistic perspective can contribute to better outcomes. For example, herbal remedies rich in polyphenols and flavonoids may act synergistically with conventional treatments to reduce oxidative stress and inflammation, key factors in skin cancer. The concept of complementary therapies in the context of skin cancer prevention involves the use of herbal remedies alongside conventional treatments to enhance overall well-being and support the body's natural defense mechanisms.

Herbal remedies, known for their antioxidant, anti-inflammatory, and immunomodulatory properties, can complement conventional therapies by mitigating side effects, boosting the immune system, and promoting overall health.

Safety Observations

As with any healthcare intervention, safety considerations are paramount when integrating herbal remedies into the prevention of skin cancer. While herbal remedies offer potential benefits, it is crucial to acknowledge and address potential risks and interactions. Safety considerations encompass the sourcing, preparation, and dosage of herbal remedies, as well as their potential interactions with conventional treatments.

Patients and healthcare professionals must collaborate to ensure that the chosen herbal remedies align with the patient's overall health status and do not compromise the efficacy of conventional treatments.

Rigorous research and adherence to quality standards in herbal product manufacturing are essential to mitigate the risks associated with variability in herbal formulations.

 Furthermore, monitoring for adverse effects and regular communication between patients and healthcare providers is fundamental to maintaining a safe and effective integrative approach. Safety considerations underscore the importance of evidence-based practice, emphasizing the need for well-designed clinical studies to evaluate the safety profile of specific herbal remedies in the context of skin cancer prevention.

The integration of herbal remedies with conventional approaches for skin cancer prevention represents a progressive and patient-centered paradigm that acknowledges the potential benefits of combining traditional and modern healthcare modalities. Collaboration with healthcare professionals ensures that patients receive comprehensive guidance, incorporating the expertise of medical practitioners into the decision-making process.

Complementary therapies embrace the synergy between herbal remedies and conventional treatments, aiming for a holistic approach that addresses the multifaceted nature of skin cancer prevention.

Safety considerations, including rigorous research, quality standards, and vigilant monitoring, underscore the importance of balancing the potential benefits of herbal remedies with a commitment to patient safety.

By navigating these concepts in a thoughtful and informed manner, individuals can embrace a holistic and personalized strategy for skin cancer prevention that integrates the strengths of both herbal and conventional approaches.

CHAPTER 8
DEVELOPING YOUR HERBAL SKIN CARE ROUTINE

One of the most important aspects of preventing skin cancer is creating a customized herbal skincare routine. The effectiveness of herbal remedies is often influenced by an individual's unique skin type, genetics, and environmental factors. Customized skin care entails knowing one's skin characteristics, such as sensitivity, oiliness, or dryness, to tailor the herbal remedies accordingly. This requires a thorough evaluation of the individual's skin health, taking into account both extrinsic and intrinsic factors, as well as age, ethnicity, and previous skin conditions.

The choice of herbs is crucial when creating a customized regimen. Different herbs have different qualities, such as being anti-inflammatory, antioxidant, antimicrobial, or photoprotective.

Combining herbs with complementary qualities guarantees a comprehensive approach to skin health. For example, calendula can be selected for its anti-inflammatory qualities, while green tea extract can offer antioxidant benefits.

Matching these herbs to the specific needs of each individual's skin improves the routine's overall efficacy. Finally, taking the season and climate into account is crucial, since skin needs can change depending on external circumstances.

An Example of a Herbal Skincare Regimen

A sample herbal skincare routine provides a useful manual for people who want to include herbal remedies in their daily routine to prevent skin cancer. It consists of applying different herbal products in a sequential manner to clean, tone, moisturize, and protect the skin.

 Cleansing can be accomplished with herbal-infused cleansers like lavender or chamomile, which remove impurities without removing the skin's natural oils. Toning can be accomplished with herbal hydrosols like rose water, which have calming and moisturizing properties.

Sunscreen is an essential component in preventing skin cancer, and herbal options like red raspberry seed oil or carrot seed oil offer natural sun protection. Developing a sample routine entails carefully considering the synergy between selected herbs, ensuring a harmonious blend that meets the individual's unique skin needs.

Herbal options such as aloe vera or jojoba oil can be chosen for their moisturizing and nourishing capabilities.

The inclusion of herbal ingredients in each step ensures a continuous supply of bioactive compounds that contribute to skin health.

Observing and Modifying

To optimize the preventive efficacy of the herbal skincare routine, it is imperative to continuously monitor and adjust it. As environmental factors and skin conditions change over time, a dynamic approach to herbal skin care is necessary.

Frequent evaluations of the skin's health, including texture, tone, and presence of abnormalities, are crucial. Monitoring also entails assessing the efficacy of the selected herbs by noting any improvements or possible negative reactions.

The selection and concentration of herbs in the herbal skincare routine are modified in response to the observed results. For example, if a person becomes more sensitive, the concentration of some herbs should be reduced or more calming alternatives should be used. Environmental shifts, like the change from winter to summer, may also require modifications in the herbal routine to address different skin needs.

Finally, keeping up with new research on the effects of herbal remedies on skin health makes informed decisions and guarantees that the routine stays current with scientific understanding.

developing a customized herbal skin care regimen requires careful consideration of each person's unique skin type as well as the careful selection of herbs. A model regimen provides a useful framework that includes cleansing, toning, moisturizing, and protecting against sun damage using herbal products. It is essential to monitor and modify the regimen regularly to maximize preventive effects and adjust to changing skin conditions. By adopting a customized herbal skin care regimen, people can promote a comprehensive and long-lasting approach to skin cancer prevention.

CHAPTER 9
FAQS REGARDING HERBAL REMEDIES FOR THE PREVENTION OF SKIN CANCER

Since skin cancer is becoming more and more common around the world, it is important to prevent it. Herbal remedies have gained attention as a potential complement to conventional methods as people look for alternative and complementary approaches. In this section, we address common questions and concerns about using herbal remedies and provide evidence-based answers to promote a thorough understanding of their efficacy.

Frequently Asked Questions and Concerns

First question: What is the efficacy of herbal therapies in preventing skin cancer?

Herbal remedies have been shown to have promising anti-cancer properties in preclinical studies; however, it is important to remember that herbal remedies should not be viewed as stand-alone preventive measures, but rather as complementary components to established sun protection strategies. Research on the effectiveness of herbal remedies in preventing skin cancer is still ongoing. Herbal compounds frequently exhibit antioxidant and anti-inflammatory properties, which may contribute to their potential preventive effects.

Question 2: In terms of preventing skin cancer, are herbal therapies safer than traditional approaches?

Herbal remedies are generally regarded as safe, but caution is still necessary when using them.

The safety profile of herbal products can differ greatly, and it is important to take into account interactions with medications or pre-existing conditions.

Conventional methods, like using sunscreen and getting regular skin exams, have a proven safety record. It is best to speak with a healthcare provider to make sure herbal remedies are safe and compatible with your skin cancer prevention regimen.

3. How trustworthy is the scientific data for using herbal medicines to prevent skin cancer?

The body of research on the effectiveness of herbal remedies in preventing skin cancer is still growing, and while some studies have shown promising results, the majority of the studies are small-scale or conducted in lab settings. Large-scale, rigorous clinical trials are required to conclusively determine the effectiveness of herbal remedies, and before making any conclusions about the preventive potential of herbal remedies, people should critically evaluate the dependability and quality of research projects.

Question 4: Should herbal remedies be used in addition to other preventive methods, or can they be employed as the only preventive measure?

To be most effective, herbal remedies should be used in conjunction with established preventive strategies. Sunscreen application, protective clothing, and regular skin screenings are still essential components of a comprehensive skin cancer prevention plan. Herbal remedies can be used as supplemental measures, enhancing the overall protective effect and promoting skin health through their bioactive compounds. However, they should not be considered the only means of preventing skin cancer.

5. Are there certain herbal therapies advised for certain skin types or risk factors?

Customizing herbal remedies for particular skin types or risk factors is still a work in progress. Different skin types may react differently to herbal compounds, and some remedies may be more helpful for people with particular risk factors, like a family history of skin cancer.

More research is needed to make personalized recommendations based on individual characteristics. For the time being, a comprehensive skin cancer prevention strategy should take a holistic approach that combines a variety of herbal remedies and conventional preventive measures.

Evidence-based Solutions

Polyphenols' Significance in Preventing Skin Cancer

Polyphenols, which are abundant in many herbal sources, have drawn attention to their potential role in preventing skin cancer. For example, turmeric contains curcumin, which has been shown in laboratory studies to have anti-cancer effects. Its ability to modulate multiple signaling pathways involved in cancer development makes it a promising candidate for skin cancer prevention. Green tea contains epigallocatechin gallate (EGCG), a polyphenol with antioxidant and anti-inflammatory properties.

Preclinical studies suggest that EGCG may help prevent skin cancer by inhibiting the growth of cancer cells and reducing inflammation caused by UV radiation.

Examining Resveratrol's Antioxidant Capabilities

Resveratrol is a polyphenol found in red grapes and other foods. It has drawn attention because of its antioxidant qualities; studies suggest that by scavenging free radicals and lowering oxidative stress, resveratrol may shield the skin from UV-induced damage. Although these results are encouraging, there aren't many clinical trials evaluating resveratrol's ability to prevent skin cancer. More research is required to determine the best amount and length of time to take resveratrol supplements to prevent skin cancer.

Inflammation and Herbal Remedies: A Protective Mechanism?

Since inflammation is a major contributing factor to the development of skin cancer, anti-inflammatory herbal remedies may be protective. Curcumin, the active compound in turmeric, has been shown in several studies to have anti-inflammatory effects; curcumin may lower the risk of skin cancer by modulating inflammatory pathways; however, putting these findings into clinical practice will require well-designed trials to confirm the safety and efficacy of curcumin and other anti-inflammatory herbal remedies in preventing skin cancer.

Herbal Research Challenges

Herbal remedies for skin cancer prevention present several challenges, including a lack of standardization and diversity of study designs that can produce inconsistent results due to variations in the concentration and composition of active compounds in herbal products. Standardized approaches to herbal research, such as the use of well-defined dosage regimens and formulations, are essential for producing credible evidence. Furthermore, collaborative efforts between herbal practitioners, clinicians, and researchers can improve the quality and applicability of research outcomes in the field of herbal skin cancer prevention.

Combining Conventional Strategies with Integration

The use of sunscreen, protective clothing, and routine skin examinations are still the cornerstones of skin cancer prevention; herbal remedies can supplement these measures by offering additional protection and promoting overall skin health. Individuals should consult with healthcare professionals to create personalized prevention plans that balance the benefits of herbal remedies with established best practices. Although herbal remedies show promise in skin cancer prevention, they are most effective when integrated into a holistic approach that includes conventional preventive strategies.

The role of polyphenols, the antioxidant qualities of resveratrol, and the anti-inflammatory effects of herbal compounds like curcumin highlight their potential benefits. Overcoming challenges in research design and standardization will be critical in establishing the true efficacy of herbal remedies. In the end, a holistic approach that integrates herbal remedies with tried-and-true conventional strategies is recommended for comprehensive skin cancer prevention. In conclusion, research on the potential benefits of herbal remedies for skin cancer prevention is exciting and has produced promising results.

CHAPTER 10
RESOURCES AND REFERENCES

When it comes to the field of herbal remedies for the prevention of skin cancer, it is imperative to have access to trustworthy sources and references. There is a wealth of information available in different formats, and choosing trustworthy sources is essential for making well-informed decisions. Several books that have been recommended can be helpful allies when learning about the fundamentals and practical uses of herbal remedies in the prevention of skin cancer. Books written by well-known authorities in the fields of dermatology and herbal medicine can give an in-depth analysis of the topic, providing insights into customs, recent studies, and possible advancements.

The websites and organizations that are devoted to herbal medicine and skin health are essential for the dissemination of current information. Reputable online platforms frequently feature bookss, forums, and expert opinions, creating a community where people can exchange experiences and knowledge. Working with organizations that are reputable in the fields of dermatology, cancer prevention, and herbal research can also help people gain a deeper understanding of the latest advancements, trends, and evidence-based practices in herbal remedies for skin cancer prevention.

Research and scientific studies are the cornerstones of evidence-based medicine. Extensive studies carried out by credible organizations have greatly advanced our comprehension of the effectiveness of herbal remedies in preventing skin cancer. Research studies that examine the bioactive components, mechanisms of action, and clinical results linked to herbal interventions are essential to read.

Peer-reviewed journals, research books, and clinical trials offer insightful analyses of the scientific foundations of herbal remedies and provide a nuanced perspective on their potential as skin cancer preventive measures.

Suggested Readings

The study of herbal remedies for the prevention of skin cancer is enhanced by the following books that are highly recommended: "Herbal Medicine: Biomolecular and Clinical Aspects" by Iris F. F. Benzie and Sissi Wachtel-Galor is an extensive resource that offers a thorough understanding of the molecular mechanisms and clinical applications of herbal medicine. In addition to providing a more general understanding of herbal remedies, this book also explores their potential role in preventing skin cancer through a holistic approach.

James A. Duke's "The Green Pharmacy" is another invaluable resource that unites traditional herbal knowledge with modern research. Duke, a distinguished botanist, provides an abundance of knowledge on medicinal plants, including those that may have the ability to prevent skin cancer. The book acts as a manual for people who want to incorporate herbal remedies into their daily routine for skin health. It highlights the significance of using nature's pharmacy to prevent and treat a variety of health conditions, including skin cancer.

The book "Herbs and Natural Supplements: An Evidence-Based Guide" by Lesley Braun and Marc Cohen is a valuable resource for dermatologists.

It offers evidence-based information on herbal remedies from a clinical perspective, providing insights into their safety, efficacy, and potential interactions. It is important for people thinking about using herbal remedies for skin cancer prevention to understand the scientific basis behind these interventions.

Websites and Establishments

Accessing the wide world of herbal remedies for preventing skin cancer can be made easier by connecting with credible websites and organizations that focus on herbal medicine, skin health, and cancer prevention. One such resource is the American Herbalists Guild (AHG), which offers a wealth of information on various herbs, their traditional uses, and new developments in the field of herbal medicine.

Herbalists, researchers, and enthusiasts can exchange knowledge and stay up to date on the latest developments in herbal medicine through this platform.

For a more targeted approach to skin health, the website of the Skin Cancer Foundation is a trustworthy information source. This organization offers evidence-based perspectives on strategies for preventing skin cancer, one of which is the use of herbal remedies.

Perusing their materials can improve one's comprehension of how to combine herbal practices with conventional dermatological methods for successful skin cancer prevention.

Being involved with the National Center for Complementary and Integrative Health (NCCIH), a division of the National Institutes of Health (NIH), guarantees access to scientifically sound information on herbal interventions for a variety of health conditions, including skin cancer prevention. The NCCIH's website provides a plethora of resources, including research updates, clinical trial information, and educational materials.

Research and Studies in Science

A wealth of research studies have been conducted to help us understand how particular herbs and bioactive compounds may help prevent skin cancer. One such study, "Anticancer Potential of Plants and Natural Products: A Review," published in the journal BioMed Research International, reviews the scientific evidence supporting the anticancer properties of various plants. It is important to investigate these thorough reviews to obtain a deeper understanding of the wide range of herbal remedies and their potential impact on skin cancer prevention.

Clinical trials that investigate the effectiveness of herbal interventions for skin health are crucial in the field of dermatology. One example of a research books that has been published in the Journal of the American Academy of Dermatology is "Herbal Medicines for the Treatment of Nonmelanoma Skin Cancers: A Systematic Review," which reviews the body of evidence regarding herbal medicines and their role in treating nonmelanoma skin cancers.

By reading through this type of scientific literature, people can evaluate the quality of the evidence and make decisions about the inclusion of herbal remedies in their skin cancer prevention regimen.

Furthermore, it is imperative to comprehend the molecular mechanisms that underlie the anticancer effects of particular herbs. "Phytochemicals as Anticancer Agents: Recent Advances in Detection, Synthesis, and Identification of Bioactive Compounds" delves into the complex biochemical pathways via which phytochemicals enact their anticancer effects. Research of this kind lays the groundwork for clarifying how herbal remedies might impede the processes that culminate in the development of skin cancer.

The three categories of references, books that are suggested reading, and scientific research provide a thorough foundation for exploring the complex realm of herbal remedies for preventing skin cancer. Through the use of reliable sources, people can arm themselves with information that is based on both conventional wisdom and modern scientific research. This approach's many facets guarantee a thorough comprehension of herbal interventions and encourage decision-making that puts skin health and cancer prevention first.

CONCLUSION

With the number of skin cancer cases rising worldwide, there is growing interest in the topic of using herbal remedies to prevent skin cancer. This thorough investigation attempts to clarify several issues surrounding the application of herbal remedies in skin cancer prevention.

Skin cancer, which includes melanoma, basal cell carcinoma, and squamous cell carcinoma, is mostly caused by exposure to ultraviolet (UV) radiation. Conventional preventive measures include wearing sunscreen, changing one's lifestyle, and getting screened regularly. However, there is growing interest in the potential benefits of herbal remedies as a substitute for or in addition to traditional methods.

Exploring these molecular pathways can offer important insights into the potential efficacy of herbal remedies for skin cancer prevention.

Many herbs have shown anti-cancer properties through different mechanisms, such as antioxidant activity, anti-inflammatory effects, and modulation of cell cycle regulation.

For example, polyphenols found in green tea have been shown to inhibit the growth of cancer cells and reduce the risk of skin cancer.

Furthermore, the significance of phytochemicals in herbal remedies cannot be overstated.

A variety of biological activities associated with phytochemicals, such as flavonoids, alkaloids, and terpenoids, have been linked to the prevention of skin cancer. These compounds function as antioxidants, scavenging free radicals produced by UV radiation, thereby reducing DNA damage and mitigating oxidative stress. Further research into the precise phytochemical composition of herbs can further our understanding of their potential to prevent skin cancer.

Additionally, one important factor to take into account is how herbal remedies affect the immune system. The immune system is essential for identifying and eliminating cancer cells.

Certain herbs, such as echinacea and astragalus, have been shown to have immunomodulatory effects, which may strengthen the body's defenses against aberrant cell growth. Researching the complex relationships between immune system function and herbal remedies can shed light on how they prevent cancer.

Sun protection is still the most important preventive measure when it comes to skin cancer. Herbal remedies that have photoprotective qualities can provide an extra line of defense against UV-induced damage. Certain herbs, like calendula and aloe vera, have been used traditionally for their calming and anti-inflammatory properties on the skin, which may help prevent sunburns and UV-related skin damage.

The discussion of herbal remedies for the prevention of skin cancer can benefit from the inclusion of cultural and traditional perspectives. A more comprehensive approach to skin cancer prevention can be achieved by integrating traditional knowledge with current scientific research. Many cultures have a long history of using particular herbs for medicinal purposes.

Herbal remedies have a lot of potential, but there are drawbacks as well. Variations in the composition of herbal extracts, problems with standardization, and a lack of clinical evidence make it difficult to determine whether they are effective. Thorough scientific research, including carefully planned clinical trials, is necessary to confirm the preventive benefits of herbal remedies and guarantee their safe and efficient use.

The investigation of herbal remedies for the prevention of skin cancer reveals a complex terrain that includes molecular mechanisms, phytochemical composition, immunomodulatory effects, photoprotection, cultural perspectives, and research challenges. Although herbal remedies show promise as a supplementary treatment, their incorporation into traditional preventive strategies necessitates careful thought and validation based on evidence. As we traverse this developing field, cooperation between researchers, medical professionals, and the general public is crucial to realizing the potential advantages of herbal remedies for the prevention of skin cancer.

From their antioxidant qualities and immunomodulatory effects to their role in photoprotection, herbal remedies offer a diverse array of potential mechanisms for preventing skin cancer. As such, they present a multifaceted approach to mitigating the risk of skin cancer.

That being said, it is important to approach these remedies with a balanced perspective, acknowledging both their potential benefits and the need for rigorous scientific validation.

Readers are encouraged to engage with this evolving field by staying informed about ongoing research and considering the potential role of herbal remedies in their skincare routines.

The journey into the realm of herbal remedies for skin cancer prevention serves as a call to explore alternative and complementary approaches to conventional strategies. The wealth of botanical resources provides a rich tapestry for investigation and potential integration into personalized preventive measures.